Introduction

Cancer is a word that always gets everyone's attention, mainly because it is something everyone tries to avoid at all cost in their lives. Not only is cancer is by all means a highly serious matter, it is a disease that destroys life - not only for the person who has the disease, but for everyone around them.

For years, chemotherapy has been the chief treatment for cancer, recommended by most medical professionals. Chemotherapy indeed has proven effective in many cases, resulting in remission and sometimes, even cure of cancer. However, there happens to be some cancer patients, as well as some medical professionals, who don't believe in chemotherapy owing to the burdens it puts on the patient's health and finances. But, what else is there for cancer patients to do?

There might be something you can try.

Not many people know this these days but nature have always had the answers to the questions that modern science has been constantly trying to find; such as the answer to cancer. If you manage to treat yourself naturally in the early stages of cancer, there is a chance you will have the chance to live a long and happy life, without having to fear and dread the consequences of cancer every single second of your life.

At the same time, by living a healthy life and using natural anti-cancer cures, you can give yourself the chance to prevent cancer as well.

This book contains a brief introduction to all-natural diet plan which will help revolutionize your dietary habits, and give you an outlook to a safe, tasty and healthy way to fight cancer, through proper nutrition and balanced diet. This book is not only about facts and research, but a personal experience too, as it contains a brief description of 10 ways my father -a cancer survivor - fought off his disease with. Moreover, this book will teach you the best possible dietary options for fighting cancer, as well as diets and recipes which have been proven successful for many other cancer patients over the years and also my own father's diet after his diagnosis with cancer.

This book, "The Cancer Fighting Cookbook: 30 day Road to Remission" will not only give you a number of recipes to choose from and try, but will also explain the science behind them. These meal plans, created by experts on cancer-related diets, will give you a number of options to revamp your entire lifestyle.

Mind it: there are a number of detoxifying recipes out there that are sometimes mistaken for anti-cancer diets. If you have tried them in the past and failed to see any improvements, it is probable that you might be skeptical of this book, as well. Let me assure you of one thing - if you will take the chance of taking full advantage from this book here, you will have the choice of different dogmatic diets to choose from. The diets described in this book have been known, in a number of cases, for producing positive results in different forms of cancer.

If you are still hesitating towards changing your entire diet plan, you are more than welcome to look up testimonials about the two revolutionary options provided in this book and just try replacing one or two meals a day with those given here. I am assure you will notice positive changes in your condition by following the guidelines provided in this book - simply by eliminating some foods from your diet, keeping your type of cancer in consideration. Your motivation and drive should also be well directed in preventing yourself from all the junk food that is offered so readily around us.

What I can also promise is that your entire way of thinking about diets and snacking will change entirely after learning all about the health benefits associated with these diet plans. After you try these diets, you will observe that they will treat your body with more gentleness and care than the regular foods that you used to eat.

These diets are not a kind of fixed prescription; rather, they are certain frameworks through which you will be able to create your very own personalized diet. Though eliminating certain foods as prescribed by these diets, you will be able to overcome your old habits of consuming additional amounts of unnecessary and harmful edibles. This book will offer you the right kind of tools that you will need to effectively eliminate your regular diets of all the foods which have been causing you trouble till now.

My book, "The Cancer Fighting Cookbook: 30 Day Road to Remission" is a result of gathered information from works of different experts and testimonials of those who have found positive results from those treatments. Here, I have provided a guideline to remove as many food allergens as possible that will produce a positive impact on your health and body vitality.

I must remind you to make sure to implement these changes as gently as possible, and to keep a constant check on your results. However, I would not encourage you to compare your results with others, because each individual has different physical conditions that come from countless other factors, besides the disease itself. I would also ask you that you realize that, the best diets for this disease would be one that helps in minimizing your immune response, which is triggered from consuming foods your body is sensitive towards. These trigger foods are different for different people, and the diet that has been most effective for someone else might not be so much for you.

There are several options in this books, but do not confuse yourself with them; rather, focus on what is best for your body keeping your personal conditions in consideration. The main idea in this book is to inspire and direct you to follow a pattern which is bound to create long-lasting changes in your entire lifestyle, if not something more concrete. Following these diets will assure you the right kind of changes your body requires to begin the healing process.

Not only facts and theories, this book actually contains real life solutions that are not only practical, but also simple to replicate. A comprehensive diet program has been explained in this book for you to adopt and try, along with different recipes to try at home. In these recipes and diet plans, you can learn about the different foods you need to consume, and the ones to avoid in your way to fight cancer.

Please remember: this book does not serve as an alternative for medical attention, no matter how sure I sound of it. I strongly advice and ask you to seek medical treatment and at the same time, follow my guidelines for a better lifestyle.

The work produced within this book is for you to use and produce a program that suits you, something that makes YOU the expert of your own body. Enjoy!

Chapter 1
Health and Wellbeing through a Vegan Diet

Most people convert into vegetarians because they feel compassion for animals; to eat meat, according to them, is cruelty to animals. Others might regard this as unreasonable, but most vegans are animal lovers, and a vegetarian diet, for them, is a way to protect animals. However, for some Vegans, their lifestyle goes far beyond animal rights. Vegans know that a vegetarian diet can guarantee them a healthy life with prevention to a lot of major diseases.

Many people misunderstand, or have misconceptions about, what a Vegan diet is all about. If you have limited or unclear idea of what a Vegan diet is, this chapter will help you get a thorough idea of what this diet entitles.

Fruits and Vegetables

Some of the main sources of minerals and vitamins are essentially fruits and vegetables, and your body requires these minerals and vitamins in order to perform its regular functions. For example, Vitamin A is required by the human body for strengthening of the immune system, and Vitamin B is needed for processing energy from food. Vitamin D is required to maintain the health of your bones and teeth. Most of these essential vitamins are primarily found in a number of fruits and vegetables. Similarly, consuming fruits with skin - such as apples and pears - are rich in fiber, which is great for maintenance of the digestive system and to enhance the health of your gut.

One huge reason that some people prefer fruits and vegetables for their daily food is their composition. Almost all fruits and vegetables are low in calories, sodium and fat; and at the same time, there is absolutely no cholesterol in them, which is amazing for people who are trying to lose weight and for people of advanced age.

Besides, high quantity of fiber present in most fruits and vegetables makes them an absolute necessity in your daily diet. Fiber helps you feel "full" without having to eat too much, and this is a reason that people with particular eating disorders are advised to include vegetables and fruits in their daily diets.

At the same time, fruits and vegetables are not "dull" as they may be considered by some people! Actually, they have the potential of filling a person with energy and stamina almost as much, or more, than any commercial energy drink. The problem with a commercial energy drink is that it dramatically boosts your energy levels for a short period of time but at the end of the high, comes a huge dip in energy that leaves you lethargic and struggling to get work done, fruits may or may not provide you the same amount of energy but in a very sustainable pace so you will have a constant stream of energy throughout the day rather than the constant highs and lows that also cause fat build up and more unhealthy conditions.

According to statistics, individuals who consume the most fruits and vegetables every day have the lowest possible risk for chronic illnesses and diseases. Moreover, their bodies are less likely to demand supplements or vitamins as their healthy diet offers sufficient nutritional value. However, this should not come as a surprise to those on a Vegan lifestyle, or to those who are aware of the benefits of a Vegan diet.

Phytochemicals

Phytochemicals are certain chemicals found in plants that are responsible for providing color, and are present in most fruits and vegetables. Nature offers us more than 12,000 phytochemicals and this is why, consumption of vegetables and fruits offer you sufficient amount of these chemicals. These chemicals are the main reason that a person who consumes adequate amount of fruits and vegetables does not need additional supplements.

Every different color of food, containing unique and different types of phytochemical, enhances the strength of your immune system, and increases its functions. I have taken the liberty to explain some of the most important ones in this chapter for your knowledge.

☐ Red Fruits and Vegetables

Carotenoids and Anthocyanins are the two main phytochemicals that can be traced in red fruits and vegetables, i.e.

- Tomatoes,
- Apples and apple by products,
- Strawberries,
- Red grapes,
- Blood oranges,
- Red cherries,
- Red onions,
- Raspberries,
- Vinegar and
- Raw apple cider vinegar

Among Carotenoid, Lycopene is the most abundantly found phytochemical found in red fruits and vegetables. This element is important for reduction of damage caused by the free radicals present in your body, and it helps in the prevention of various physical problems in the body, such as,

- Heart diseases,
- Prostrate issues,
- Cancer, and
- Skin damage caused by the sun.

These red fruits and vegetables aid your memory function, and help to maintain your urinary tract health, as well as your heart. They also contain high levels of Vitamin C which promote cellular renewal process in the human body.

☐ Orange Fruits and Vegetables

Orange fruits and vegetables also consist of Carotenoids which have DNA repairing properties, and help in the prevention of heart diseases, a number of types of cancer, along with strengthening your vision. Besides, orange foods offer you appropriate quantity of Vitamin A and Potassium which help in keeping your skin and eyes healthy, and provide protection against blood infections.

Orange fruits and vegetables are also high in Vitamin C, for example,

- Pumpkin,
- Carrots,
- Apricots,
- Cantaloupe,
- Mango,
- Nectarines,
- Oranges,
- Papaya,
- Persimmons,
- Peaches,
- Tangerines, and
- Butternut Squash.

☐ Yellow Fruits and Vegetables

Yellow foods are known for their high composition of Antioxidants and Vitamin C, which is helpful in maintenance of gums and teeth. The yellow Phytochemicals in these fruits and vegetables help enhance your body's healing power, along with improvement in mucus membranes.

Some other benefits of yellow fruits and vegetables include:

- Faster absorption of iron,
- Prevention of inflammation,
- Improvement of circulation, and
- Prevention of heart diseases.

A lot of the benefits of yellow foods tend to overlap with the ones provided by orange fruits and vegetables, such as,

- Yellow apple,
- Yellow figs,
- Lemons,
- Yellow kiwi,
- Pineapple,
- Yellow pears,
- Summer squash, and
- Bananas.

☐ Green Fruits and Vegetables

The phytochemicals found in green fruits and vegetables include Sulforaphane and Indoles, both of which are helpful in the prevention of cancer. Moreover, they help in improving your circulatory system, since they tend to consist of high levels of Vitamin B and other minerals. These green fruits and vegetables are also highly rich in Vitamin K, which is responsible for improving your vision, and in the maintenance of bone and teeth.

The relatively yellower green vegetables consist of Carotenoids Lutein, along with Zeaxanthin composition, which helps in the prevention of cataracts. Besides, these types of green fruits and vegetables have been known to prevent osteoporosis.

Most common green and yellow-green fruits and vegetables that are consumed widely include,

- Seaweed,
- Kale,
- Broccoli,
- Avocado,
- Green grapes,
- Honeydew melon,
- Kiwi,
- Limes,
- Green pears,

- Artichokes,
- Arugula, and
- Asparagus.

☐ White Fruits and Vegetables

Strong phytochemicals, known as Allicin and Allium, are found in some white fruits and vegetables, which are responsible for creating an environment in your body which is anti-bacterial, Anti-fungal and anti-viral. These kinds of foods help in prevention of heart diseases and some forms of cancer.

Some of the common fruits and vegetables that are a part of our daily diet are,

- Chives,
- Mushrooms,
- White pear,
- Garlic,
- Ginger,
- Fennel,
- White peaches,
- Green onions, and
- Jerusalem artichoke.

White fruits and vegetables have the potential to bring your cholesterol levels down, because most of them contain about zero calories.

☐ Fruits and Vegetables of Other Colors

Fruits and vegetables that consist of other colors - i.e. purple, blue or indigo - consists of anti-aging properties, and are loaded with antioxidants. Anthocyanins and Phenolics are the two most important antioxidants found in such foods.

There are certain foods which consist of high levels of vitamin C as well, which help in blood circulation and prevent blood clots in the heart. These types of foods are extremely helpful in improving memory, and maintaining a healthy urinary. The different fruits and vegetables of this nature that we consume regularly, or should consume, are,

- Blackberries,
- Blueberries,
- Purple cabbage,
- Eggplant,
- Raisins,
- Purple grapes,
- Prunes,
- Figs,
- Black currants,
- Elderberries, and
- Plums.

Nutrition

Besides the important vitamins and minerals, the wide selection of fruits and vegetables that are a part of a Vegan diet offer a whole array of other nutrients.

☐ Reduced Saturated Fats

The meat and dairy products that a non-vegan diet allows make us consume large quantities of saturated fats. Fruits and vegetables, on the other hand, help reduce the amount of saturated fats consumed, leading to a better health. In particular, our cardiovascular health is improved tremendously through this.

☐ Carbohydrates

Carbohydrates, found in a number of fruits and vegetables, are essential for providing energy to the human body.

☐ Fiber

Vegan diets are high in fiber, which prompts healthier solid discharges, and effectively helps battle against colon disease.

☐ Magnesium

Supporting in the retention of calcium, Magnesium is an ignored vitamin in significance to a solid eating regimen. Nuts, seeds, and dim verdant greens are a great source of magnesium.

☐ Potassium

Potassium equalizations water and causticity in your body and invigorates the kidneys to release the poisons. Weight control plans high in potassium have demonstrated to lessen the danger of cardiovascular infections and growth.

☐ Folate

This vitamin is an imperative part of a solid eating regimen; Folate assists with cell repair, creating red and white platelets and metabolizing amino acids.

☐ Antioxidants

For assurance against cell harm, cancer prevention agents are one of the most ideal approaches to help your body. Numerous analysts additionally accept that cell reinforcement helps protect your body against shaping a few sorts of a tumor.

☐ Vitamin C

Other than boosting your immune system, Vitamin C helps keep your gums sound and helps your wounds mend speedier. It is also a well-known cancer prevention agent.

☐ Vitamin E

Vitamin E is advantageous for your heart, skin, eyes, and cerebrum; it may even help keep Alzheimer's disease away. A diet rich in grains, nuts and dull verdant greens is brimming with Vitamin E.

☐ Phytochemicals

Plant-based foods give phytochemicals, which help to keep and mend the body from the tumor, support defensive chemicals, and work with cell reinforcements in the body.

☐ Protein

Most Americans eat an excess of protein, but mainly in non-Vegan diets, i.e. red meat, which is not as beneficiary as people hope it to be. Actually, beans, nuts, peas, lentils and soy items are better source of protein that is a good approach to get the perfect measure in a vegan diet.

Chapter 2
Vegan Diet Plan: Meals and Recipes

It is not easy to think of starting a Vegan Diet, and to actually implement one in your lifestyle could be a challenge, especially if you are someone who loves their red meats and animal proteins.

This is exactly what this chapter is all about - helping you in adopting a healthy Vegan-diet that is practical and not as difficult as one might believe. Instead of going through the hassle of coming up with an entire plan on your own, you will be able to put into use this easy-to-imitate plan, and ensure effective results quickly.

However, I do suggest that you consult your doctor first before trying this diet and customize this meal framework further to suit your physical condition, as well as follow the restrictions that your doctor might put you on.

A Vegan diet follows these main frameworks:

For Breakfast

You can consider the following food items for your breakfast every day:

- Porridge or cereal with soy and rice or nut milk and fresh fruit;
- Scrambled tofu with grilled tomatoes and mushroom on toasted English muffin;
- Toast with Marmite or avocado and jam or baked beans;
- Fresh fruit salad and soy yogurt;
- A simple fruit smoothie;
- A few muffins; or
- Vegan pancakes with maple syrup.

For Lunch

The following items can be consumed for a perfectly vegan lunch diet:

- Minestrone soup with crusty bread;

- Vegetable Frittata;
- Tempeh or bean burger;
- Hearty salads using lentils or beans, potatoes, rice or pasta;
- Sandwich or wrap by using a variety of salads, mustard, hummus, roasted vegetables, vegan mayonnaise, falafel, crispy tofu, mock meat slices or vegetable schnitzels;
- Vegan sushi; or
- Baked potato topped with mixed bean and veggie salad.

For Dinner

The following suggestions are perfect for a delicious dinner for your vegan diet:

- Vegetable sausages with garlic mashed potatoes, green beans and gravy;
- BBQ tofu or veggie skewers with corn on the cob;
- Vegan lasagna, and some spaghetti bolognaise;
- Vegetable curry, or roti and daal;
- Mixed vegetables stir-fry with tofu;
- Tempeh or nuts served with rice or noodles;
- Mushroom risotto; and
- Chili non-carne with mixed green salad.

For Snacking

Who doesn't realize the importance of snacks? You need at least something to munch on when food cravings attack! Not just any snack would do for these occasions; rather, there are some amazing snacks to control those little hunger pangs.

- Fresh fruit is perfect for all occasions;
- Raw vegetable sticks dipped in hummus, salsa or guacamole;
- Raw almonds or other nuts;
- Pumpkin seeds (pepitas) or other seeds;
- Soy yogurt;
- Wholegrain crackers, such as Ryvitas or Vitawheats, with toppings are good for instance fresh tomato, avocado and Marmite;
- Rice cakes with peanut butter or Tahini and baby spinach leaves, which are entirely fresh;

- Dates and other dried fruit;
- Fruit Cups;
- Raw Bliss Balls;
- Baked beans, preferably salt-reduced;
- Glass of fortified soymilk in which you have the option of trying to blend with fresh fruit in order to create soy smoothie high in nutrition; or
- A glass of green smoothie.

When you want to Treat Yourself

Of course you would want a break from the mundanely healthy diet now and then; if you are craving for something sweet, these following foods are perfect considerations.

- Blueberry muffins;
- Banana and Walnut muffins;
- Raspberry and White Chocolate muffins;
- Vegan sweets or desserts and cakes;
- Licorice;
- Muesli bars in which you should make sure to check the label to assure no usage of animal products;
- Sesame Snaps; or
- Vegan chocolate.

Easy to Create Recipes

If you are not wholly satisfied with this simple diet framework, or if you are interested in experimenting with your grocery list, here are some easy-to-create recipes which will offer you good options for you vegan diet plan.

These recipes have been created by experts and loved by all those looking to survive Hashimoto's just like you through a vegan auto-immune diet plan. These recipes offer a good range from smoothies and salads to a variety of main courses. You will never find vegan recipes boring or dull anymore. Enjoy the bursting flavor and healthy nutrition in the following.

If you have ever thought vegan recipes dull or unappetizing, these will definitely change your mind!

Raw Green Smoothies

These recipes below are designed for four adults in large portions; it is very easy to moderate the recipes to depending upon the number of people at hand.

For Pineapple/Blackberry Green Smoothie

- 24 ounces of water
- 8 or 16 ounces of blackberries
- 4 ounces of pineapples *(Peeled from the outer skin; there is no need for you to core in case of a high-speed blender. Chop in smaller chunks to add to blender)*
- 1 orange, *peeled and seeded*
- 2 full stems of mint green, *with leaves*
- 1 bunch of chard
- 3 tablespoon dulse
- 8 dates, *pitted (These are added for sweetness and are optional)*
- 2 tbsp. chia seeds

For Banana Beet Green Smoothie

- 32 ounces of water
- 3 medium-sized bananas
- 2 tbsp. Mace powder *(optional)*
- 5 dates, *pitted*
- 1 Bunch of beet greens
- A handful of spinach *(Optional)*
- 2 tbsp. of chia seeds

Banana Pineapple Green Smoothie

- 32 ounces of water
- 1 medium-sized banana
- 4 ounces of pineapples, *peeled from the outer skin*
- 2 full stems of mint green, *with leaves*
- ½ bunch of chard
- 1 handful of parsley
- 5 dates, *pitted (optional)*

Raw Soup Recipes

These recipes are meant to serve at least four to five people. You can adjust the quantity used of each ingredient accordingly depending upon the number of people.

☐ <u>Corn Bisque</u>

Ingredients

- 12 ounces of warm water
- 32 ounces of corn, *frozen*
- 2 cloves of medium-sized garlic
- Himalayan salt, *to taste*
- Pepper, *to taste*

Preparation

- Blend all the ingredients until they are smooth.
- Pour these into a large bowl.
- Add the corns and enjoy warm.
- If you are looking for an extra crunch, add a handful of sunflower seed.

☐ <u>Corn Chowder</u>

Ingredients

- 16 ounces of water, *warm or hot*
- 32 ounces of corn, *frozen*
- 2 cloves of medium-sized garlic
- 1 tbsp. of cumin, *ground*
- Himalayan salt, *to taste*
- Pepper, *to taste*

Ingredients, Part-II

- 1/3 medium-sized jicoma root, *cut in a food processor to look like rice*
- ½ green bell pepper, *chopped into small cubes*
- 16 ounces corn
- 2 medium-sized avocados, *cubed*

Preparation

- Blend all the ingredients mentioned in the first part of the ingredients.
- Pour the mixture into a large bowl.
- Mix in the all the ingredients of Part-II.

☐ **Taco Raw Soup**

Ingredients

- 28 ounces of water, *warm or hot*
- 2 Roma tomatoes
- 2 stalks of celery
- 6 tbsp. of corn
- 2 medium-sized carrots
- 2 springs of green onion, 2 ounces of white onion
- 1 handful of cashews
- Few springs of parsley
- 1 clove of garlic
- 1.5 tbsp. of chili powder
- ½ tbsp. of cumin
- ¼ tbsp. of white or black pepper
- 1 tsp of Kirkland organic seasoning
- Himalayan salt, *to taste*

Garnish

- 3 medium-sized avocados, *cubed*
- 2 Roma tomatoes, *cubed*

Preparation

- Blend all the ingredients together in a blender.
- Pour the mixture into a bowl.
- Add the garnish on top, and serve.

☐ **Green Salad**

Ingredients

- Mixed spring greens, *chopped*

- Cherry tomatoes, *chopped*
- Cucumber, *sliced*
- Lemon, *juice and zest*
- Spices and salt, *for garnish*

Preparation
- Mix all the ingredients together.
- Add spices, lemon juice and salt according to your taste.

Gluten Free Recipes

☐ <u>Gluten-free Salad</u>

Ingredients:
- Spinach
- Romaine lettuce
- Cilantro
- Onions
- Tomatoes
- Zucchini

Procedure:

Mix to serve. You can add corn chips with salsa as well.

☐ <u>Gluten-free Salsa</u>

Ingredients:
- 5 medium-sized tomatoes
- 1/4 onion
- Handful of cilantro
- 2 cloves of garlic
- 1/2 medium-sized bell pepper
- Salt, *to taste*

Procedure:
- Chop the vegetables thoroughly but without turning them into absolute mush.
- Mix all the ingredients in a bowl and serve.

☐ **Hummus**

Nothing is more appetizing than a bowl of hummus topped with delicious, fresh herbs and sun-dried tomatoes, or with fresh tomatoes and pine nuts. You can also use it as a spread on bread, or with lettuce leaves, or add it to soups.

☐ **Parsley Salad**

Ingredients:
- A handful of Parsley
- Cilantro
- Green onions
- Dill, *chopped into small pieces*
- Tomatoes, *chopped*
- Cucumber, *chopped*
- Sesame
- Hemp seeds
- Salt, *for seasoning*
- Lemon juice, *freshly squeezed*
- A few garlic cloves, *smashed*

Preparation:
- Mix all the ingredients together.
- Season with salt and juice.
- Add the cloves of garlic for a more spicy taste.
- Let the salad sit for about fifteen minutes before serving.

Main Course

For your main courses to go with appetizers there are a number of choices as well.

☐ **Borsch Soup**

This soup is just way too good for you to not try. If you're a soup lover then prepare to meet a new favorite.

Ingredients:

- 16 ounces of fresh beets, *chopped*
- 16 ounces of carrots, *chopped*
- 16 ounces of cabbage, *chopped*
- 1/2 tsp salt
- 1/2 tsp dill weed
- 16 ounces of onion, *chopped*
- 32 ounces of broth, *beef or vegetable*
- 1 16-ounce can of tomatoes, *un-drained and diced*
- 1/4 tsp of pepper

Directions:

- Combine the beets, onion, carrots and broth in a large pan.
- Bring to a boil.
- Reduce the heat and cover the pan.
- Let it simmer for about thirty minutes.
- Add the cabbage and tomatoes.
- Cover the top and let it simmer for about thirty minutes.
- Try stirring it in salt, pepper and dill.
- Use sour cream for topping each serving.

☐ **Vegan Pizza**

Of course, Vegans have the option of making amazing pizza just as much. You can even use vegan cheese in your pizza or substitute it with tofu which is crumbled and firm.

For the Dough:

- Start off by reducing water volume to about 12-14 ounces. Make sure to prepare it using the dough cycle in case of a bread maker.

Preparation:

- After the bread is ready, divide it into two equal parts.
- Roll out the dough into circles or stretch it with your hands.
- Preheat your oven to 400°F.

- Lay out the dough on baking sheets.
- Spread the sauce on top.
- Spread the cheese over the sauce.
- Add the toppings.
- Bake for about 5 minutes using the bottom rack.
- Bake on the top shelf for 5 more minutes until it becomes golden brown.
- Keep the pizza on top rack for the very last 30 to 40 seconds.

Possible toppings:
- Pineapple
- Apple, *thinly sliced*
- Bell peppers
- Red onions
- Tomatoes
- Zucchini
- Mushrooms

For Drinks

You can make peach iced tea for your drink as it will complement the variety of flavors of your dishes.

For Dessert

☐ Rhubarb Tart

The vegan Rhubarb tart is an absolute wonder in terms of desserts. You can serve it with coconut vegan ice cream as well.

Ingredients:
- 48 ounces of rhubarb, *chopped*
- 1 tsp of cinnamon
- ½ tsp of cardamom, *ground*
- 3 ounces of wheat flour
- 8 ounces of berries of your choice
- Zest of 1 orange, *grated*

- 6 ounces of cane sugar, *unbleached*

Topping:

- 8 ounces of wheat- or white-flour
- 4 ounces of oats
- 4 ounces of pecans, *sliced and crumbled*
- 6 ounces of brown sugar
- A pinch of salt
- 2 ounces of olive oil

Preparation:

- Preheat the oven to 375°F.
- Oil a large baking dish, or several individual dishes.
- Toss all the ingredients together in a bowl until a good coating is achieved.
- Transfer this to a prepared baking dish.

Delicious Vegan Dishes
Simple Recipes to Replicate at Home

☐ Vegetable Biryani

Ingredients:

- 15 ounces of basmati rice
- A pinch saffron threads
- 2 ounces of cashew nuts, *roughly chopped and roasted*
- 2 tbsp. vegetable oil
- 1 cauliflower, *cut into florets*
- 2 medium-sized potatoes, *cut into chunks*
- 4 ounces of red lentils
- 4 ounces of French beans, *trimmed and cut in half*
- A handful of curry leaves
- 2 handfuls of peas, *frozen*
- A small bunch of coriander
- 1 tsp cumin, *ground*
- 2 tbsp. vegetable oil
- 1 small green chili, *chopped*

For the paste:

- 1 large onion, *roughly chopped*
- 1 large ginger, *roughly chopped*
- 5 garlic cloves
- 2 tsp of curry powder

For the carrot salad:

- 4 carrots
- A pinch of golden caster sugar
- Lemon, *freshly squeezed*
- A handful of cashew nuts, *roughly chopped*
- A handful of coriander leaves, *roughly chopped*
- A thumb-sized ginger, *shredded into matchsticks*
- 1 tsp cumin seed, *toasted*

Direction:

- Soak the rice for about 30 minutes and rinse.
- Add saffron and cover the pan to boil.
- Stir once and then turn the heat off.
- Leave for 10 minutes and stir again.
- Leave it covered.
- Mix all the other ingredients using a food processor.
- Heat oil in a pan; add the paste followed by cauliflower and potatoes.
- Keep cooking and add green beans and lentils.
- Cover it with 400ml of water.
- Add in salt and curry leaves.
- Let it simmer for 20 minutes; add peas in last 2 minutes.
- Stir in rice and serve.

Add sugar and lemon juice to the carrots by sprinkling. Add other ingredients as well, and serve with the biryani.

☐ **Vegetable curry**

Ingredients:

- Vegetable oil
- 4 ounces of mushrooms, *quartered*

- 1 medium-sized red pepper, *diced*
- 1 medium-sized red onion, *peeled and chopped*
- 1 courgette, *diced*
- ½ medium-sized butternut squash, *peeled and diced*
- 6 ounces of cauliflower, *broken into florets*
- 600 ml of curry-based sauce
- 400 ml water

Method:
- Fry onions in vegetable oil for 10 minutes in a pan.
- Add other vegetables in and stir.
- Add your curry sauce and let it simmer for about 25 minutes.
- Add water if sauce gets thick.

Chapter 3
The Paleo Approach

The Paleo approach goes beyond just a diet; it also explains our prioritization of sleep and management of stress, along with protection of circadian rhythms. This diet also incorporates some mild and moderate activities in our daily routine.

Following the Paleo diet will create good impacts in your life, provided you keep these factors going as well. People with autoimmune diseases should especially consider adhering to this diet very seriously. A very important part of Paleo diet is to completely eliminate processed food from your diet, as well as gluten.

Moreover, you would need to completely avoid the following foods in Paleo diet:

- Eggs, and egg whites in particular
- Nuts
- NSAIDS, i.e. Aspirin
- Seeds
- Nightshades
- Foods that are Gluten cross-reactive
- Alcohol
- Fructose (more than 20 kg each day)
- Emulsifiers
- Nonnutritive sweeteners
- Additives and
- Thickeners.

There are some reasons you should avoid these foods, because:

- They cause irritation of gut
- They cause gut dysbiosis, which is basically overgrowth of the gut
- They act as adjuvant which stimulate the immune system
- They act as carriers of molecules in the gut,
- They increase permeability of the gut, and
- They cause inflammation.

There are some evidence that suggest it is hormonal birth that has the potential to contribute to digestive hormone deregulation and hunger, which ultimately leads to inflammation of immune system. Consumption of a nutrient-dense diet is the most important factor of this entire approach. Increased risk of autoimmune diseases is directly associated with micronutrient deficiencies. In case of an autoimmune disease, you are highly likely to experience deficiency of:

- Fat soluble vitamins of A, D, E, K
- Mineral, such as iron, copper, zinc, magnesium, iodine and selenium etc.
- Vitamin B and C
- Non-vitamin nutrients, such as CoQ10
- Antioxidants
- Omega-3 or, fatty acids
- Amino acids, such as glycine,
- Fiber.

While you have to eliminate the aforementioned foods you must also focus on increasing your consumption of some of the following foods:

- Cruciferous vegetables such as kale, cabbage, arugula, broccoli, turnips, cauliflower, watercress, Brussels sprouts and mustard greens etc.

- Organ meat and offal, as least five times a week.

- Fish and shell fish, especially the wild ones, which should be taken at least three times a week.

- All sorts of vegetables, taken at least eight to fourteen cups each day.

- All green vegetables.

- All kinds of fruits of colors, as well as colored vegetables.

- All sea vegetables, excluding algae.

- Quality meats from grass-fed, wild and pasture-raised animals.

- Quality fats from pasture-raised and grass-fed animal fats, as well.

- Sweet fruits, maintaining fructose intake to twenty grams.

- Probiotic foods, such as water kefir, coconut, kombucha, coconut milk, yogurt.

- Glycine-rich foods, such as organ meat, joints/skin and bone broth.

You should consider improving your intake of trace minerals as well by opting for dirty sea salt or Himalayan Pink salt. You have the option of eating organic produce to create a good difference. Make sure to drink plenty of water in between your meals.

Try consuming the vegetables and fruits raw or cooked. Try including at least something green in each meal. Reserve the high sugar and dried fruits for your occasional treats.

Points to Consider

- You can opt for a low Fermentable Oligo Di Monosaccharides and Polyols (FODMAP) approach in combination with your autoimmune diet, provided that you have confirmed Small Intestinal Bacteria Overgrowth (SIBO).

- Insoluble fiber helps in prevention of inflammation, and reduces your chances of getting C-reactive protein, as well as reduction of cancer risks, and those of cardiovascular disease. It has the potential of reducing bile acid loss and is highly essential for ghrelin suppression, after you have consumed your meals. You can add digestive support supplements to your diet if you find intact pieces of fiber in your stool. Try limiting your diet to cooked vegetables till your overall digestion is improved.

- There is no scientific explanation for the exclusion of goitrogenic vegetables by those with thyroid disorders. It is in fact only a myth.

- People tend to avoid fruit due to its high content of sugar, which is a correct decision in case of FODMAP-intolerance. However, there is an endorsement for fruit in moderate amounts. These are rich sources of vitamins, fiber, minerals, and antioxidants. In general, you have the option of enjoying at least two to five servings of fruit on a daily basis.

- Remember that your intake of Omega-3 is critical; therefore, you should try to consume at least 1:1 to 1:3 ratio of Omega-3 to Omega-6. This can be maintained naturally by consuming pasture-raised and grass-fed meat along with fish and poultry of the same kind. In the case of additional consumption of conventional meat, you must focus on increasing the overall intake of oily cod-water fish like mackerel, herring, salmon, kipper, sardines, trout, carp, fresh tuna, and anchovies.

- Protein intake is also highly critical. You have the choice of healing your body through foods which are animal based to shellfish and fish. Fish and shellfish contain the kind of protein which tends to be relatively more digestible compared to meat- and plant-protein.

- Vegetables are important, as well. You must not even consider skimping on vegetables! If you a type of person who have trouble consuming large vegetables servings and smoothies, you can opt for a little amount as part of your daily meals. If you have gastrointestinal issues in digestion, you can consume digestive support supplements in addition to your meals. Try limiting your diet to cooked vegetables in the beginning as well.

Other Pointers

These foods can be reintroduced after improvement is achieved in a stabilized form:

- Egg yolks,
- Legumes,
- Walnut oil,
- Grass-fed ghee,
- Macadamia nut oil, and
- Gluten free alcohol.

The following foods should only be taken in moderate amounts:
- Coconut butter,
- Coconut cream concentrated,
- Creamed coconut,
- Coconut flakes,
- Fresh coconut,
- Coconut chips,
- Carob,
- Rooibos tea,

- Black and green tea,
- DGL,
- Apple cider vinegar,
- Wine vinegar,
- Balsamic vinegar,
- Coconut water vinegar,
- Coconut water,
- Vanilla extract, if cooked,
- Pomegranate molasses, and
- Maple syrup.

The following foods should only be consumed occasionally:

- Maple sugar,
- Honey, very occasionally,
- Dried fruit,
- Dates and date sugar,
- Molasses, and
- Unrefined cane sugar, which includes sucanat, evaporated cane juice, muscovado, and coconut amino.

It is recommended that you should opt for larger meals, which should be further apart. Try transitioning to this new diet slowly; your intermittence should not be fast in case of an autoimmune disease. Try avoiding excessive liquid with your meals and remember to chew the food thoroughly. Try avoiding meal intake within two hours of bedtime because it might cause disruptions in your sleep cycle.

Some Useful Supplements

- Digestive enzymes,
- Plant enzymes,
- Pancreatin,
- Ox bile,
- Betaine HCl,
- L-glutamine,
- Fermented cod liver oil,
- Magnesium,
- Vitamin C,
- DGL,
- Prescript-Assist Probiotic supplement, and

- Collagen.

Never undermine the critical significance of enough sleep and stress management. Make sure to protect the circadian rhythms and try avoiding bright lights at night time. Nurture your social connections and make sure to have fun and relax.

The Paleo Diet Plan

Similarly to the Vegan Autoimmune Diet Plan, the Paleo diet plan also suggests you come up with a customized plan by consulting with your nutritionist or your doctor, in general. These professionals would have the right amount of information about your health and conditions, which will enable them to make better decisions for you.

A simplified framework is provided in this book in order to ease you into this diet. Don't hesitate to mix it up with your own ideas, or to add and modify recipes when necessary, whilst remaining in the boundaries of the diet.

Drinks

- The Maple Pumpkin Collagen Shake is an amazing way to boost your energy. This drink is perfect for an early morning jump start as well.

- The Natte Pumpkin Spice is a crowd pleaser. Everyone loves a spiced pumpkin drink, and this drink provides them just that with only a healthier version of what they desire.

Appetizers and Condiments

When it comes to appetizers and condiments, the following are suggested:

- Citrus-spiced cranberry sauce! Who doesn't love cranberry sauce? The recipe by Bre'anna is perfect as a side dish and it offers an amazingly spicy combination without going overboard with any of the ingredients.

- The Asparagus Bacon-Wrapped by Holly and Raj is just a classic! The dish is yummy and simple.

- The Sweet Potato Crisps by Mary are perfect when it comes to instant hunger pangs feeding. These are not only simple to make but also a great pleaser of your little ones.

Sides

- Sweet Potato, Artichoke, and Bacon Soup is a recipe which works amazingly with the elements of chunkiness and creamy texture. This is a perfect holiday meal recipe and is a crowd favorite if you add bacon to it.

- Apple-Cranberry Holiday Stuffing by Mickey of Autoimmune Paleo is another option for delicious sides. Sides become rather needed in times of holidays and this autoimmune friendly dish is good enough to feed a large number of people.

- The Maple-syrup-delicata-squash by Elise of Simply Recipes, is an all-seller. The dish is sold on its name as well as the mention of maple and Brussels sprouts are more than enough for most people. The dish is scrumptious and has a beautiful look to it as well owing to the contrasting colors.

- Honey Balsamic Roasted Carrots by Samantha of Sweet Potatoes and Social Change is another valid option. The carrot and honey recipe is quite easy to make and is a definite crowd pleaser. The pop in this dish is created through the usage of rosemary and balsamic.

- Herbed Whipped Parsnips by Rach of Meatified is a recipe bound to simply melt in your mouth. The parsnips tend to come out with additional buttery texture and oh so very creamy which you are definitely going to enjoy. No one is going to miss the mashed potatoes as long as you serve them this amazing dish.

Main Dishes

- Baked Fresh Ham by Sarah of The Paleo Mom is a heavy meal dish. This is enough to fulfill your requirements of having large meals in good ample amounts. Ham is considered a good way to go by many out there when it comes to your main course. You have the option of using herbs such as thyme and rosemary along with spices such as cinnamon and ginger as well instead of the seed based spices mentioned in the recipe.

- Roasted Lamb Ribs with Garlic and Parsley by Jo of Comfort Bites Blog is a favorite of all those not in favor of ham. You have the option of making lamb which a favorite protein for many. The recipe offers a perfect combination with recommended side dishes. It won't hurt to slightly spice it up by moving away from the traditional dishes of ham.

Desserts

- Hibiscus Ginger Gummies by Sophie of A Squirrel in the Kitchen is known for pleasing the crowd. These are perfect when you are looking to prepare something before time. Your kids are going to love them and the fun recipe will keep the entire family quite happy throughout the day.

- Fresh Ginger Spice Cookies by Bethany of Adventures in Partaking is another dessert option you can go for. Who doesn't crave a homemade cookie? It becomes more of a necessity in your holidays in particular. You will end up making batches of these autoimmune friendly cookies solely based on the taste and aroma.

- Rustic Pear Galette by Gabriella of Beyond the Bite appears to look scary in terms of replicating it. You are required to enjoy the entire cooking process by taking your time. You will find this recipe easy to make once you get a hang of it.

- Pumpkin Roll with Cinnamon Molasses Spread by Alaena of Grazed and Enthused is a recipe that offers a perfect treat for your holidays and snack times. The right amount of sweet is achieved through the cinnamon molasses spread.

Chapter 4
Diet Suggestions for Adrenal Fatigue Recovery

One side effect is common in all type of cancer, and that is adrenal fatigue. Cancer, even when treated, not only affects a patient's body, but also their psychology and mental stability. Along with depression and gloominess, the body is quite likely to experience adrenal fatigue syndrome or chronic tiredness, which is almost inevitable in all form of cancer.

What is Adrenal Fatigue?

Adrenal Fatigue is also referred to as Adrenal Fatigue Syndrome. Here, the word 'syndrome' suggests a combination of more than few indicators and symptoms. This particular syndrome can be described, in simple terms, as 'Underperformance of your adrenal glands'.

This is actually a disease that is caused by stretched or intense stress. However, this particular disease is not limited to stress alone, but also as a cause of chronic infections, like bronchitis and pneumonia, in particular. The paramount symptom, as the name of the disease suggests, remains excessive fatigue.

In case of Adrenal Fatigue, the kind of fatigue faced by a person should not be confused with usual tiredness. Rather, this fatigue is characterized as a state of tiredness which is not relieved through means of sleep or rest, or any other means. Adrenal fatigue is not easily identifiable, specifically due to its normality, which is common in a modern lifestyle.

The tricky part is that you may even behave and appear as normal as possible, without any apparent indicators of physical ailment. Yet, you might have a generally tired state all the time. People suffering from Adrenal Fatigue Syndrome are usually seen dependent on caffeine and similar stimulants in order to wake up or to make it through the day.

The syndrome has been referred to in the past as:

- Non-Addison's Hypoadrenia,
- Neurasthenia,
- Sub clinical Hypoadrenia,
- Adrenal neurasthenia, or
- Adrenal apathy.

Conventional medicine usually fails to formally recognize adrenal fatigue despite its commonality around the globe. This symptom has the potential of creating havoc in your life. In serious cases, the adrenal glands exhibit such limited activity that the person fails to even get up for more than few hours in a day. The disease also affects coordination and functioning of each organ of your body. With reduction in adrenal functioning, the systems in the human body are extremely affected. Some of the common areas that experience change include:

- Carbohydrate metabolism
- Fat metabolism
- Protein metabolism
- Fluid and electrolyte balance
- Cardiovascular system
- Sex drive
- Heart

There are many other forms of alternations that occur on both cellular and biochemical levels as a compensatory reaction for the reduction in adrenal functioning. The body tries its best to restore balance and to make up for the underperformance of adrenal glands but a lot of damage is done during this process.

Causes of Adrenal Fatigue

Adrenal Fatigue is caused when the adequate demand of stress is not met by the Adrenal glands. The mobilization of your body responses to all kinds of stresses is ensured by adrenal glands, namely physical, emotional and psychological stress.

Adrenal glands assure stabilization of your body through the release of hormones. These hormones cope with stress through regulation of energy production and storage in the body, as well as in regulating heart rate, muscle tones and the immune system.

Regardless of the nature of your stress - either because of the death of a loved, or the daily stress of your life - the adrenal glands are responsible for coping with them. In case of any adequacy, you fall victim to adrenal fatigue syndrome. Your glands might not stop functioning, but they will fail to maintain the optimal level of output. The reason for this is over stimulation which, in intensified stress or chronic situations, has the ability to over stimulate the glands.

Who is likely to become susceptible to Adrenal Fatigue?

Everyone has the possibility of experiencing Adrenal Fatigue at one point or other in their lifetime. Even the healthiest person can become susceptible to this disease in case of a crisis or continuous stress, which can completely drain your adrenal glands. However, there are certain factors which have the potential to make you relatively more vulnerable to this disease, such as,

- Poor diet,
- Extremely little sleep,
- Highly reduced rest,
- Intensified pressure,
- Substance abuse,
- Chronic illness,
- Repeated infections,
- Bronchitis/pneumonia,
- Prolonged bad relationships,
- Poverty,
- Imprisonment,
- Stressful job, and
- Gestation.

Commonality of Adrenal Fatigue

There are no formal data statistics available for recent analysis for Adrenal Fatigue. Dr. John Tinterra, a specialist in low adrenal function, estimated an approximate through his experience in this particular field. He suggested that almost 16% of the general public can easily fall into the category of suffering from severe adrenal fatigue; also, this percentage could rise up to 66% if the low cortisol was factored in as well. However, these statistics were estimated before the stressful 21st century, and therefore would be much higher these days.

How to Identify Adrenal Fatigue?

Everyone feels fatigued one time or more during the day, but it is advised that you don't go about diagnosing yourself after reading all the symptoms. Rather, you should conduct a doctor for a formal diagnosis. There are certain noticeable factors that can help you diagnose your condition:

- Experiencing tiredness without any apparent reason,
- Experiencing difficulty in getting up in the morning even with sufficient sleep,
- Feeling overwhelmed,
- Having difficulty in recovering from stress or physical illness,
- Continuous craving of sweet and salty edibles, and
- Feeling most energetic and alert after 6 PM.

Health Conditions Relating to Adrenal Fatigue

A lot of demands are placed on the adrenal glands in serious physical illnesses, such as cancer. This can make Adrenal Fatigue a severe and chronic symptom, like arthritis and morning tiredness.

Medical treatments that inculcate usage of Corticosteroids always create a high reduction of adrenal function. The corticosteroids are designed specifically for imitation of actions, performed by the adrenal hormone known as Cortisol. Basically, the need for Corticosteroids arises majorly in situations where your Adrenal glands are unable to produce the demanded quantity of Cortisol.

Can people with adrenal fatigue return to normal?

It is absolutely possible for people experiencing adrenal fatigue to feel normal at times, when the right kind of care and caution is provided. You can always consult your doctor to help you out of this disease while considering your specific bodily needs.

Symptoms and Indicators of Adrenal Fatigue

As the name suggests, fatigue is the primary symptom of Adrenal Fatigue Syndrome. This disease basically leads to reduced production of hormones in the body which are critical for just about everything. This contributes to the diversity present in every other case of adrenal fatigue. There are common symptoms and indicators but each case tends to present itself in a somewhat unique manner.

The symptoms of Adrenal Fatigue can be divided into two categories: the most commonly experienced symptoms and the rare and less common symptoms.

☐ Common Symptoms

Difficulty Getting Up Every Morning

Amongst the primary causes of adrenal fatigue is insufficient sleep, and increasing the number of hours for sleeping is one of the most effective means to recovery. However, it is common for people suffering from adrenal fatigue to wake up feeling extremely tired even after a long sleep. There are few factors to be held responsible for this: significant stress in early stages of this disease creates high levels of Cortisol and adrenaline in human bodies, which keep people alert at all times. This state of continuous alertness hinders natural sleep cycles and results in prevention of restful sleep.

Later stages of adrenal fatigue are characterized by relatively lower Cortisol levels. However, there is an abnormal pattern when it comes to blood sugar level. People suffering from later stages of adrenal fatigue tend to experience lower blood sugar levels in the morning. This is why many patients with adrenal fatigue have habit of late night snacking.

Continuous High Levels of Fatigue

The later stages of adrenal fatigue make it difficult for the glands to assure sufficient production of the hormones. This results in lower production levels of Cortisol, Adrenaline and Norepinephrine.

The lack of such critical hormones in a patient's body helps explain their inability to get up in the morning, or their having no energy to last the day. However, it is quite common for sufferers of Adrenal Fatigue to experience energy regain at night.

Inability to Cope with Stress

Those suffering from adrenal fatigue experience difficulty in dealing with different forms of emotional and physical stress. This is another contributing factor to their persistent state of tiredness, along with a diminishing function of adrenal glands. When a person faces a stressful situation, their body automatically becomes dependent on adrenal functioning for release of a number of hormones. Their internal strength, awareness and focus are enhanced significantly.

However, in case of adrenal fatigue and reduced release of hormones, the patient fails to respond in this manner, these results in lack of enthusiasm along with a state of disinterest, anxiety, irritability, craving for salty food, etc.

Mineral and fluids are excreted from your body by the kidneys. This regulatory process is carried out primary by two hormones: Mineralocorticoid and Aldosterone. An integral part of the adrenals is responsible for the production of these two hormones. When your adrenals experience continuous fatigue, they offer reduced production of Aldosterone, which results in significant excretion of valuable minerals through urine. Those with exhausted endocrine systems tend to experience frequent urination which is characterized by age but can actually be a consequence of depleted Adrenal glands.

As a result of this, those suffering from Adrenal Fatigue lose their ability to maintain balanced levels of important minerals in the blood, including sodium, magnesium and potassium. This is the reason behind your body craving for salty foods - as replacement of the lost potassium. If you experience such sudden cravings, you might just be experiencing Adrenal Fatigue.

Higher Energy Levels at Night

You can feel devastated in terms of your energy levels when your body fails to produce the required amounts of Cortisol needed. In case of a healthy individual, highest levels of Cortisol are produced early in the morning, and have a tendency to decline as the day progress. In case of sufferers of adrenal fatigue, however, energy reaches its peak in the evenings. A patient experiences tiredness throughout the day, followed by sudden energy at night. Earlier stages of Adrenal Fatigue offer such symptoms when your glands still have the capability of producing significant levels of Adrenaline and Cortisol.

An Undermined Immune System

Our immune system takes help from the anti-inflammatory effects provided by Cortisol. Most people are not aware of the fact that inflammation is usually an indication of your body fighting a certain kind of infection; Cortisol keeps a check on the entire process. This increases the importance of maintaining a sound level of Cortisol production in the body for your health. In case of elevated levels of Cortisol during intense stress, the anti-inflammatory effects gain strength and become more intense than needed. This, in turn, affects your immune system and prevents it from functioning normally.

This weakened state of immune system can last as long as the stress lasts, exposing your body to diseases due to vulnerability. Conversely, in case of low Cortisol production, your immune system tends to offer exaggerated reactions to pathogens which lead to chronic inflammation. Moreover, multiple respiratory diseases are caused by the very same reason, as well as some auto-immune disorders.

A person's condition is entirely dependent on the stage of their disease. The early stages of this disease are characterized by suppression of immune system due to exaggerated levels of Cortisol, followed by increased vulnerability to infections. Later stages of adrenal fatigue encompass low-level production of Cortisol, leading to chronic inflammation and different allergies. Neither one of these situations is a good one.

Other Symptoms

Many of the symptoms of Adrenal Fatigue are in direct link with the aforementioned symptoms as well. Here is a list of symptoms that you might experience depending upon your stage:

- Asthma,
- Allergies,
- Respiratory complaints,
- Lines in your fingertips,
- Loss of muscle tone,
- Dark circles,
- Dizziness,
- Dry skin,
- Low sex drive,
- Lower back pain,
- Numbness in your fingers,
- Poor circulation,
- Extreme tiredness,
- Frequent urination,
- Joint pain,
- Low blood pressure,
- Low blood sugar, and
- Weight gain.

Your defense against adrenal fatigue starts from the kind of food you consume. The idea behind creating a diet plan to support your adrenal glands is to revitalize your life and regain your true productivity levels.

Two aspects have to be considered in this case. Firstly, there are certain foods that you must avoid in order to prevent your adrenal fatigue from worsening. Secondly, there are certain foods that you must actively consume to boost your recovery process.

Such a diet requires you to have fixed and appropriate timings for all three meals during the day, as well as consumption of nutritious foods. You must avoid consuming any foods that your body is intolerant or sensitive to.

Identification of Food Allergies and Intolerances

Food intolerances are something to understand and pay attention to if you suffer from Adrenal Fatigue. These sensitivities basically prevent absorption of useful nutrients, as well as promote inflammation. This, in turn, disturbs your sleep cycle. Moreover, these prevent your gut from proper digestion and excretion. This is why, the first indicators of food intolerances are constipation and diarrhea, along with other gut-associated issues.

Optimal digestion is hindered in allergies and intolerances, which ultimately result in lowering your energy levels. This also promotes growth of harmful bacteria in your gut, which weakens your immune system. You can deal with the intolerances quite simply by implicating the rules described here.

- Avoid that particular food completely. If you can clearly identify the food which is creating issues for you, then you must forget about it instantly, no matter how much you like it. If you are confused, you can try out avoiding each food at a time to find out what's troubling you. This will help you clearly point out your allergies and intolerances.

- You can opt for supplements for strengthening your gut. The most commonly consumed supplement is Glutamine which helps out in repair and regeneration of your intestinal lining. Give licorices a try as well, in order to protect your intestinal lining from irritants.

- You can consume supplements for digestion improvements in case of symptoms like constipation, gas or bloating. Digestive enzymes are helpful in this case as they allow you to digest with more ease.

Dietary Principles

Most cases of Adrenal Fatigue have a history of processed foods and unnecessary sugar. In order to recover, you must change your dietary habits, first and foremost. Here are certain guidelines that you should follow for a speedy recovery:

- **Eat at the Right Time**

It is very common for people nowadays to exhibit unhealthy eating patterns. Breakfast, despite its importance, is usually skipped followed by a light lunch, and a heavy evening meal. You must instantly alter this if you don't want to worsen your situation. Never underestimate the importance of breakfast, especially for those suffering from adrenal fatigue.

Your body requires the right amount of fuel in order to last the entire day. Your breakfast must be rich in protein, as well as contain a small amount of carbohydrate. A good example of such breakfast is a vegetable omelet paired with blueberries. The second option is a healthy smoothie. Additionally, you must avoid sugar-based cereals and other traditional breakfast elements, i.e. waffles, pancakes, etc.

Maintaining optimal sugar level in the blood is a struggle for Adrenal Fatigue patients. This is why three meals are suggested in a day, with appropriate intervals.

- **Foods to Consume and Avoid**

There are certain foods that can be labeled as super foods, owing to their contribution in Adrenal Fatigue. You must consume them, keeping the following basic guidelines in consideration.

- Reduce your sugar consumption and opt for low-sugar fruits.
- Consume more protein throughout the day.
- Prefer coconuts, seeds and avocado, as well as dairy products for fats.
- Cut out caffeine; give up your morning tea or coffee. If you struggle to wake up try a cold shower, it's better for your skin and cardio health.

- Always keep your body hydrated. It is more important for adrenal fatigue sufferers. You can even add little amounts of sea salt and lemon in your water as well as most patients consist of electrolyte deficiencies as well.

Super Foods

At the same time, there are some "super foods" that are going to speed up your recovery process, as described below.

o **Bone broth**

Bone marrow is an extremely important nutrient that helps your immune system. You can consume this by making a simple broth with bone marrow, known for creating a reduction in inflammation and boosting of the immune system. It encourages healthy cholesterol as well, and offers essentials like minerals, amino acids and vitamins for easy absorption.

o **Seaweed**

Seaweeds offer phytonutrients and minerals in rich quantity. These nutrients are hard to find in normal diet plans, but are delicious when added to a salad or stir-fried.

o **Fermented drinks**

Fermented drinks are extremely helpful for your digestion. However, this does not mean beer, but rather some fermented drink that you can make at home or purchase from food stores. These offer a rich quantity of minerals and a boost of healthy bacteria that will create improvement in your digestion. Kvaas and Kombucha are two effective fermented drinks.

The Adrenal Fatigue Recovery Diet

Here's a simple list of guidelines to follow for your Adrenal Fatigue recovery diet:

- You should start primal, i.e. a Paleo diet.

- Make sure to have sufficient breakfast. Your breakfast should have, at the very least, 40 grams of protein. Also, try consuming your breakfast within 30 minutes of waking up to balance out your Cortisol levels.

- Consume unrefined salt; don't use processed salt, rather opt for sea salt or Himalayan salt.

- Never skip a meal; eat regularly.

- Try consuming your carbohydrates in the form of fresh vegetables and fruits.

- Don't go overboard with drinking water. Eight glasses of water per day should be enough for your body's needs. Too much water has the ability to cause an imbalance of sodium in your blood.

- Eat healthy fats like coconut oil, grass-fed animals and egg yolks.

- Avoid a low-carbohydrate diet, and opt for starchy vegetables and fruits.

- Say no to caffeine and alcohol.

- You can consider Adrenal Fatigue recovery supplements, which include:

  - Adrenal glandular treatment,
  - Herbal adrenal support,
  - Vitamin C,
  - Pastured chicken and beef, and
  - DHEA.

Chapter 5
Adrenal Friendly Food Recipes

☐ Quinoa Tabouleh

Quinoa is an extremely beneficial grain for your body - a super food on its own. This grain serves as an amazing source of vegan protein. It is comprised of a number of rich materials, namely:

- Dietary fiber
- Vitamin B6
- Iron
- Thiamine B1
- Folate
- Magnesium
- Riboflavin
- Phosphorus
- Copper
- Zinc
- Manganese

Tabouleh is very easy to assemble, and can be consumed as a simple snack or properly served for lunch or dinner. The recipe provided in this book allows you to personalize the dish in accordance with your taste preferences. You can add a number of other ingredients like chickpeas, scallions, cucumber, lemon juice or jalapenos to spice this dish up.

Ingredients:
- 8 ounces of quinoa, *dry*
- 4 ounces of parsley, *thinly chopped*
- 2 ounces of coriander, *chopped*
- 2 ounces of mint leaves, *severed*
- 2 medium-sized tomatoes, *diced*
- 4 tbs. of olive oil
- Salt, *to taste*
- Pepper, *to taste*

Instructions:

- Start by adding two cups of water and bring it to a boil.
- Stir in the quinoa into the boiled water.
- Make sure to reduce the heat to low and keep stable for about 15-20 minutes or until the water is reduced.
- In the meantime, prepare all the other ingredients and keep them near.
- When the water is reduced, use a fork to full the quinoa, and let it cool.
- After the quinoa has cooled down, mix in all the other ingredients gently.

☐ **Roasted Beet Salad**

Betaliain is a natural pigment in beets that adds the extra vibrancy in its color. This pigment is an excellent and powerful antioxidant. Consumption of betaliain in beets is not only good for your internal systems, but also for your skin. Beets are significantly rich in folate, manganese, copper, fiber, potassium and magnesium.

Ingredients:

- 2-3 medium-sized beets
- 1/2 inch strips of one-seeded red pepper
- 1 large-sized tomato, *cut into one-inch cubes*
- 1 small-sized red onion, *finely sliced*
- 3 cloves of garlic, *peeled and thinly sliced*
- 1 small block of feta cheese, *cut into cubes*
- 1 tbs. sesame seeds, *for topping*
- Green/black olives, *chopped*

Instructions:

- Scrub the beets in water first, and cut them into one-inch cubes. Do not peel them.
- After having gathered the ingredients, start the cooking process by pre-heating your oven to 350°F or 180°C.
- Rubbing the cubed beets with olive oil.
- Space them out on a baking sheet.

- Place these beets in the oven for approximately 20 or until they become tender.
- Roasting the red pepper and the sesame seed on the stove while the beets are being roasted in the oven.
- Add the beets, garlic, red onion, red pepper, tomato along with the cheese in a bowl and mix gently.
- Add the sesame seed and mix gently one last time.

If you're looking for a presentation idea, try mixing the juice of one medium-sized lemon, one finely chopped garlic clove, parsley and tablespoon of extra virgin olive oil. Add salt and pepper for taste, as well.

☐ **Mixed Bean Salad**

Beans have always been regarded as magical in myths and fairy tales. In reality, this is quite true, as well. Bean are a significant source of vegan protein, and they consist of significant levels of essential minerals and vitamins, including thiamin, niacin, manganese, Vitamin C, Riboflavin and Magnesium.

Ingredients:
- Beans
- 1 clove of garlic, *finely chopped*
- 2 tsp of olive oil
- 2 tsp of lemon juice, *freshly squeezed*
- 1 stalk of celery stalk, *finely chopped*
- 1/2 red pepper
- 2 ounce of black olives, *chopped*
- 2 ounces of parsley leaves, *chopped*
- A handful of Arugula leaves
- 1/2 small-sized red onion, *thinly sliced*
- Salt, *to taste*
- Pepper, *to taste*

Instructions:
- This recipe works best if you use a mixture of beans instead of one type. Beans are acceptable in the form of a canned mix as well. For a good mix look for a

combination of black-eyed peas, black and garbanzo beans along with kidney beans.

- Roast the red pepper, if you prefer them that way. To add more texture to the dish you have the liberty of using your own choice of grain, pasta or rice according to your preference.
- Gather all the ingredients together.
- Start by placing the lemon juice in a jar with olive oil and garlic. Shake it well to mix.
- Add the rest of your ingredients in a bowl.
- Add your mixed dressing in and toss very gently to ensure proper mixing.

Chapter 6
Setting Right Our Hormonal Balance

Falling into the pits of depression is quite common for cancer patients, as well as natural. If motivational speeches and "Hang in There, Kitty" posters don't cheer someone up, it is time to get up and get on the road to recovery. One way to do his is through bringing a complete change in your food and diet plans to battle depression.

There are some special foods that help not only in people suffering from depression due to cancer, but anyone with depression. Actually, it is a person's hormonal imbalance that is one of the major cause of depression, which can be helped with some hormonal reset recipes!

Reset recipes

Below you are going to find some simple and easy-to-make recipes which can help you in balancing your hormones. We will elaborate different types of recipes which are going to cater to a complete fitness regime.

☐ <u>**Grain-Less cookies with Almonds:**</u>

Ingredients:

- 16 ounces of almond flour
- 3½ tbsp of flaxseeds, *ground*
- ½ tsp of baking soda
- 1 pinch of sea salt
- 1 pinch of black pepper, *freshly ground*
- 3 tbsp of maple syrup, *pure*
- 2 tbsp of coconut oil
- 1 large pinch of cinnamon, *ground*
- 1 dash of vanilla extracts
- 1 tbsp of sesame seeds, *roasted*

Instructions:

- Start you cooking by preheating the oven to 350°F.
- Next, prepare two cookie sheets with parchment paper.
- In a big bowl, combine all the almond flour, sea salt, ground flaxseeds, a pinch of black pepper and baking soda, and mix together.
- Add maple syrup, coconut oil and vanilla extract.
- Mix them all together until the mixture becomes dough.
- Add the cinnamon and the sesame seeds. Mix them together until they blend properly.
- Transfer multiple scoops of the dough on the baking sheets, in small scoops so that they are not too big, but the size of a spoon.
- Bake for 15 minutes or until all the cookies have turned golden in color.
- Remove the cookies from oven, and keep them aside to cool down.

☐ Gluten-free, Dairy- and Sugar-Less Raspberry-and-Lime Tarts

Ingredients:

- 1 tart crust, *raw*
- 32 ounces of nuts (pecans, walnuts, almonds), *raw*
- ¼ tsp of sea salt
- 3 ounces of dates, *pitted*
- ½ tsp of cinnamon
- 12 ounces of cashews, *soaked in water for 3 hours*
- 3 ounces of almond milk, *unsweetened*
- 4 ounces of lime juice, *freshly squeezed*
- 4 tbsp of maple syrup, *pure*
- 2 ounces of virgin coconut oil
- 1 Pinch of sea salt
- 12 ounces of organic raspberries, *fresh*
- Topping of your choice
- Cashew Filling
- 1 small lime, *zest only*

Instructions:

- Soak the mixed nuts in water for at least 3 hours, and set it aside.
- Coat a muffin tin with coconut oil, and keep aside, as well.
- Blend all the nuts together with sea salt, dates and cinnamon until the mixture becomes dough.
- Scoop the mixture into each of the muffin cavities; use your hands to mold the shape.
- Transfer the pan to the fridge.
- Rinse the cashews in water, and drain; pat them dry.
- In a food processor, add the cashews with almond milk. Puree together until smooth.
- Add the lime zest, pure maple syrup, lime juice, sea salt, raspberries and coconut oil. Puree until smooth.
- Remove the crusts from where you kept it in the fridge and spoon in the mixture.
- Transfer the filled crusts back into the fridge, and chill for another 6/7 hours.
- Remove from fridge before serving; serve by topping with fresh raspberries.

☐ **Triple-Layered Vegan Sandwich**

Ingredients:

- 4 slices of whole-grain bread, *gluten-free*
- 4 Table spoons of hummus
- 1 table spoon of hot sauce
- 1 cup mixed greens such as spinach and arugula
- 4 Table spoons of cooked white beans
- 1 thin sliced small apple
- 1 small pear, thinly sliced
- ½ small cucumber, thinly sliced
- ½ small carrot, shaved
- sea salt and pepper depending upon your taste
- pinch of chili powder
- 1 box of Campbell's Organic Tomato & Basil Bisque

Procedure:

- Toast the bread, if you like your bread toasted.
- Spread hummus and hot sauce on the surface of each slice of bread. Top two sliced with greens, beans, apple slices, cucumber slices, pear slices, shaved carrot, sea salt, and pepper. Now, add a dash of chili powder depending upon how much you like it.
- Place the other two bread slices on top of the toppings and slice both sandwiches in half and set them aside.
- Pour bisque into a small pot over medium heat and cook it until it gets warm which is going to take about 5 minutes. Transfer it to two serving bowls and serve warm with the sandwiches and enjoy the delicious snack.

☐ Gluten-free Cherry Oatmeal Cookies

Ingredients:

- 8 oz gluten-free rolled oats
- 2 ounces of flaxseeds, *ground*
- 3 tbsp of raw pumpkin seeds, *shelled*
- 2 tbsp of chia seeds
- 6 tbsp of almond butter, *slightly melted*
- 3½ tbsp of honey
- ¼ tsp of vanilla extract
- 3 tbsp of dried cherries, *chopped*
- 1 pinch of sea salt
- 1 large pinch of fresh orange zest
- 1 pinch of cocoa powder or cinnamon

Instructions:

- Take a large bowl and combine oats, flaxseeds, chia seeds, pumpkin seeds and mix them well. After mixing, set it aside.
- Meanwhile in a separate bowl, combine slightly melted almond butter, vanilla extract, and honey.
- Mix them well to combine properly and transfer it to the oat mixture.

- Mix them both well.
- Add dried cherries, sea salt, and orange zest and then add cinnamon or cocoa powder.
- Roll the mixture into small balls which should be about 1 inch in diameter.
- Place them in the fridge until ready to serve.

☐ **Sweet potatoes and kale soup**

Ingredients:

- 3 tbsp of extra-virgin olive oil
- 1 large Vidalia onion, *diced*
- 1 large fennel bulb, *thinly sliced*
- 1 large garlic clove, *minced*
- 2 small fresh sage leaves, *finely chopped*
- 1 head curly kale, *finely chopped and stems removed*
- 1 large red bell pepper, *finely diced with stem and seeds discarded*
- 2 large sweet potatoes, *peeled and cut into pieces*
- 2 large carrots, *diced*
- 32 ounces of Pacific Foods Chicken Bones stock
- 8 ounces of organic fresh corn kernels
- Sea salt, *to taste*
- Black pepper, *freshly ground*
- A large dash of chili powder
- A dash of red pepper flakes, *freshly ground*
- 2 tbsp of pumpkin seeds, *for garnish*

Instructions:

- Heat extra-virgin olive oil in a large heavy stock pot over medium heat.
- Add the onion, fennel bulb slices, and minced garlic.
- Reduce heat to low and cook until it becomes tender.
- Keep stirring often.
- Add fresh sage, sweet potatoes, chopped kale, diced bell pepper and diced carrots.
- Add some corn and broth or stock.
- Bring it to a boil over medium heat and cover.

- Reduce heat to a simmer for around 25-30 minutes or until vegetables are tender.
- Add sea salt, pepper, crushed red pepper flakes and chili powder.
- Transfer it to the serving bowls and serve warm.
- Garnish with pumpkin seeds.

☐ **Quinoa cranberry salad**

Ingredients:

- 8 ounces of quinoa
- 1 red bell pepper, *finely diced*
- 3 tbsp. of dried cranberries
- 2 tbsp. of raw cashews, *chopped*
- 2 tbsp. of fresh basil, *finely chopped*
- 2 tbsp. of balsamic vinegar
- 2 tbsp of olive oil
- 2 tsp of orange juice, *freshly squeezed*
- ¼ tsp of fresh orange zest
- Sea salt, *to taste*
- Pepper, *to taste*

Instructions:

- Cook quinoa according to the directions are given on the package.
- Take a big bowl and toss the cooked quinoa with bell pepper, cashews, cranberries, and basil.
- Take a small bowl and whisk vinegar, orange juice, olive oil, orange zest, sea salt, and pepper.
- Drizzle it over the quinoa salad and it is ready to serve.

☐ **Strawberry apple Paleo crumble**

Ingredients:

- 16 ounces of organic strawberries, *halved and stems removed*
- 2 to 3 chopped organic apples
- 8 ounces of almond flour

- 2 ounces of coconut oil
- ¾ tsp of vanilla extract
- A pinch of cinnamon, *ground*
- 2 tbsp. of Stevia, *in raw baked form*
- 4 tbsp. of almonds, *sliced*
- ½ tsp of fresh mint leaves, *finely chopped*

Instructions:

- Preheat the oven to 375°F.
- Prepare an 8 x 8-inch glass baking dish.
- Spread a small amount of coconut oil and the berries and apples.
- Combine almond flour, vanilla, coconut oil, cinnamon and Stevia in a separate bowl.
- Mix the dough to create a crumbly consistency.
- Add more almond flour; if needed then sprinkle this crumble mixture over the fruit in the baking dish.
- Bake for 30 minutes or at least until it turns golden brown and tender.
- Top with sliced almonds and mint.
- Serve warm.

☐ **Black bean and Tahini dip:**

Ingredients:

- 1 15-ounce can of black beans, *drained and rinsed*
- 2 ounces of tahini, or sesame seed, *paste*
- 1½ tsp of flax seeds, *ground*
- Sea salt, *to taste*
- Pepper, *to taste*

Instructions:

- In a food processor, combine all the ingredients together, and puree till s smooth mixture surfaces.
- Transfer the mixture to a serving bowl.
- Serve chilled.

Best Times during the Day to Eat

Yes, it is important to know what to eat and what to avoid staying strong and healthy is very important but at the same time, it is also very overpowering factor knowing *when* to eat. Actually, the time when you are consuming a food item is just as much important as the quality of the food. Rather, it is equally important to keep you away from perpetual sickness.

Our mothers kept telling us how important breakfast is, but there are only a few of us who actually listened. Did you listen and have a proper breakfast? Chances are you didn't believe Mom because that's what everyone does. However, as we grew up, we learnt of the importance of a hearty meal in the morning, and how it can help your body to get ready for the day to come. Another bigger and more important advantage of breakfast is that it is capable of bringing down the chances of coronary illnesses, diabetes and obesity.

We may be only talking about breakfast here, but that does mean that it is the only important meal of the day. No, you are not allowed to skip any other meal just because you have had a proper breakfast. The rest of the meals are equally important for maintaining proper health.

☐ Morning

The first and most important advice that anyone can give you about your eating habits would be to have a good breakfast every morning. As per a report published by the American Heart Association, analysts have contemplated the wellbeing results of 26,902 male health experts whose ages varied from 45 to 82, which is more than a 16-year period. After consulting with the statistics they concluded that the men who skipped breakfast had a 27% higher chance of heart attacks or passing away from coronary illness, than the individuals who made sure that they take their breakfast regularly.

As indicated by the researchers, skipping breakfast will not bring you any good and will definitely not assist you in losing weight if that's the delusion you have.

We have already explained in detail how it is extremely important for our body to get proper nutrition in the morning. Otherwise, you are likely to suffer from grave hormonal disorder. There is an increased chance that staying hungry in the morning will make you even hungrier later on, and you will be craving food to the extent that you will eat whatever comes to you. You will be more inclined to eat bigger portions at lunch and dinner. This is really not going to go in your favor because it is going to prompt a surge in the blood glucose levels.

It is always a bad idea to starve yourself at one point followed by taking in a lot during the next meal, such cases of sudden sugar rush can invite in diabetes, hypertension and elevated blood cholesterol levels - all of which are danger figures that can eventually turn in to a heart attack. Hence, you need to be very careful when it comes to not skipping your breakfast.

Now that we have established the fact that eating in the morning is very important, the next question is: *what should you eat?* This is a question that is critical for setting your glucose levels for the rest of the day. For the sake of discussion, let's say that you eat something that is entirely grain and has some fat and protein, so that your glucose is going to rise and go down gradually. This is exactly the kind of pattern we are looking for.

On the other hand, if you eat something refined, i.e. an excessively sweet cinnamon roll - it is the worst thing you can eat. The reason why it is very harmful to your body is because your blood glucose levels will spike all of a sudden, and then drop too low you will get hungry again very soon. You would want to eat more and more junk food; even if you keep on feeding your body, you will feel hungry.

In order to give your body a more reliable glucose pattern, you should try some cereal, but the ones made up of whole grain. Otherwise, it won't have a good impact on your body. Among other food options, you can have a wheat-bread toast with almond margarine, or an omelet filled with spinach and avocado. One of the most filling breakfast options would be a sweet potato, with a smidgen of cinnamon and a little bit of margarine.

Who says you need to eat only grains in the morning? You can have whatever you want to as long as it is healthy and does not make you crave anything else.

☐ Afternoon

It is very important for you to fill yourself up with the right amount of energy. After you have taken a breakfast, you might need a small snack in the afternoon that should fulfill your energy. You must have heard your elders telling you this a lot of times: *"Eat your breakfast like a king, lunch like a prince and dinner like a beggar"*.

Why do you think that is? It would make sense because if you power up your body early in the morning, your body will rely on that throughout the day. This is why it is very essential to make sure that you provide yourself with enough energy in the morning so that it keeps you going throughout the day. That is the reason why in numerous European nations, the biggest meal of the day is the breakfast. Preferably, you need to give yourself energy before you start the day.

In case you are accustomed to eating a little meal for lunch and a bigger supper later, you can still do that by treating yourself with a generous feast that has essentially fewer calories but is large in volume. For example, you can have a large bowl of fruits and raw vegetables that is not going to be very high in caloric measure, but has essentially all the nutrients that you need.

☐ Evening:

Don't go too hard on yourself! Calories get consumed regardless of when you eat them; so hypothetically, there should be no problem in eating them for dinner also. The problem here is that if you have an overwhelming supper, you're not as capable of disposing of those calories before you go to bed because by the end of the day, there will hardly be any activity left for you to do.

What you don't blaze off is more prone to be put away as fat, as you turn out to be less dynamic toward the end of the day, says Tracy Lockwood, a registered dietitian at *F-Factor Nutrition*. Eating excessively near sleep time expands your glucose and insulin, which makes you have some major difficulty in sleeping properly.

It has been confirmed by a lot of the scientists that people who eat right before are bed are generally more obese also. The reason behind this is that one; they are unable to wear all that fat off. Because they get fat, the level of Cortisol in their bodies also increases a great deal, which later leads to more obesity.

Two, late eaters make frequent visits to the fridge, and consume a lot of sweet treats, i.e. frozen yogurt and ice creams, chocolates, etc. These foods can make the glucose levels sore really high just before bed and can, at the same time, lower levels of hormone melatonin, which should help you feel drained.

As you can see, it is the hormonal disturbance that is causing the problem. An energy boost that originates from your supper, which may have comprised of pasta, rice or bread, can go about as a brief stimulant, making you feel more wakeful quickly after a feast. Additionally, it is not prescribed to rest quickly after a meal - particularly a major one - since it increases your chance for indigestion. After a large fatty meal, you can even experience acid reflux. In order to get rid of all these problems, you are advised to walk a little after taking your meal. This way you will be able to stay slim, and there will be no chance for acid reflux. *Keeping it light is the key factor that you need to remember!*

In European countries, it is a practice to eat late, but they are not overweight. That is due to the fact that Europeans are used to walking, all through the day and at night, and especially after a very fatty and overwhelming dinner.

There's unmistakably no recipe for adhering to a good diet that applies to everybody for keeping up a healthy weight and staying away from the disease, yet paying consideration on *both* what and when you eat may be a decent place to begin.

Chapter 6
Ten Natural Cancer Treatments

There are many ways in which you can treat your cancer so don't lose hope just yet. Try these treatments known to have produced effective results for cancer patients across the globe. The ten natural cancer treatments for cancer are explained in details in this chapter.

1. Juicing and Garson Therapy

This is a natural treatment for cancer which is based on the following essentials:

- Coffee enemas,
- Organic foods,
- Beef liver,
- Raw juices, and
- Natural supplements.

This therapy is actually based on revitalizing the human body's natural healing abilities. There are absolutely no damaging side effects associated with this therapy. The human immune system is boosted up with energy to fight against cancer along with degenerative diseases like heart disease and arthritis.

The therapy has different elements for various purposes. For instance; coffee enemas are meant for detoxification. Your body is kept stress free and detoxified from all kinds of toxins. Following are some of the natural supplements included in this remedy:

- Lugol's solution,
- Potassium compound,
- Pancreatic enzymes,
- Vitamin B-12, and
- Thyroid hormone.

2. The Budwig Protocol

Replacement of your fatal processed oils and fats with natural fatty acids leads to the rejuvenation of your cells. According to Dr. Budwig's research, consumption of a mixture of flaxseeds, cottage cheese, and flaxseed oil provides the best results of rebuilding and rejuvenation of the human body cells.

Cottage cheese is highly rich in saturated fats and sulfur protein whereas flaxseed is filled with electrons. The amazing combination of these elements leads to easy assimilation and absorption of the aforementioned vitals by the human body.

3. Proteolytic Enzyme Therapy

Pancreatic Proteolytic Enzymes are the true representation of the human body's primary defense against cancer. A therapy of such is high on protein and bases itself on consumption of a holistic diet for the creation of a sound environment. This is the perfect environment to trigger the self-healing process of human body.

4. Chelation-Based Vitamin-C Therapy

Chelation therapy is based on usage of natural compounds and chemicals for the elimination of poisonous metals from the human body. The therapy is known for having anti-oxidizing effects for very long periods of time. The patients can consume edibles with high levels of Vitamin C along with this therapy in order to fight cancer or prevent it altogether.

5. Essential Oil Therapy with Frankincense

Dr. Budwig has also recommended usage of Essential oil to fight against cancerous tumors. This therapy is known for its effectiveness in eliminating cancer. The treatment has been proved effective in the following kinds of clinical treatments:

- Brain cancer,
- Colon cancer,
- Breast cancer,
- Pancreatic cancer,

- Stomach cancer, and
- Prostate cancer.

The oil basically helps in regulation of cellular epigenetic functions which in turn causes the genes to trigger self-healing processes.

6. Probiotic Supplements and Foods

Probiotics are certain microorganisms which are known for promoting a naturally high balance in the intestinal microflora. These foods and supplements enhance your digestive functions along with the absorptions of miners. A leaky gut can be healed with their consumption. All of these processes ultimately help in preventing cancer. You can consume Probiotic foods like cheese and kefir for this therapy.

7. Sunshine and Vitamin D3

You can keep your body healthy and cancer-free as long as you have the support of fat-soluble vitamins and minerals in it. Vitamin D3 has been suggested as a huge help owing to recent research studies. The biggest source of this vitamin is natural sunlight whereas you have the option of taking supplements as well.

8. Turmeric

Turmeric is amazing is stopping cancer in the tracks and its effectiveness is particularly high for treatments of breast cancer, skin cancer and colon cancer.

9. Oxygen Therapy

The major cause of cancer is regarded as the deficiency of oxygen. This leads to creation of an acidic environment in the body. Cancer cells are anaerobic in nature. This clearly means that cancer cells cannot survive in an environment with high levels of oxygen. The oxygen therapy is based on this very same principle.

10.   A change in Routine

Everyone has routines throughout their lifetime but having a healthy routine that has been designed around your alertness levels in the day will help change your body rhythm. For example, try doing 10-30 pushups every morning, as soon as you slap your alarm off, get to the group and complete 3 sets of 10 push up for beginners , the next day try squats or burpees or planks but ensure that the routine you've picked pushes you to give a little extra. Try sending your kids to school or work, try taking a cold shower instead of a hot one. The idea is to try new things and to feel the rush of life once again as we change our boring old routines.

Conclusion

By now, you have been enlightened with the knowledge of all the benefits of healthy and nutritional diet plans. You are well aware of the process required to achieve well-being and perfect health through diet alone. You have been warned about different health related issues that are associated with dairy, in order to make you realize the importance of a vegan diet as an alternative.

The information related to different diseases, states and disorders and their connection with nutrition will help you realize the power of food and natural remedies. You can fully identify what is right for you and how to make your choices.

In this book, you have been offered all the right incentives to start your journey towards a healthier life. You have all the necessary equipment and information to regain your natural health. The documented effects and facts should have made you realize the existence of people similar to you out there.

If these people have the potential to change their entire lives, then so do you. The positive effects on your mental health have been noted down for you in order to provide you with a complete insight into the benefits offered.

Different aspects of a vegan lifestyle have been highlighted along with an array of different diet options for you. Your body can thrive only through utilization of natural means and remedies. The delicious food recipes which have been offered to you are not only simple to understand but equally easy to replicate. There's nothing stopping you now from achieving your perfect lifestyle and desired health.

To be honest, the book is called "The Cancer Fighting Cookbook: 30 day Road to remission" but my father, within 14days of implementing these changes, already reached a stage where his blood work showed, he no longer had any sign of cancer, but the doctors refused to give him remission status until he finished his cycles of Chemotherapy and frankly, the Chemotherapy hurt him more than his stage 4

Lymphoma did and the doctors gave an estimate of 40 days of lifespan left, where they even predicted that Chemo couldn't save him, Chemo DID help my father initially though! The lymph node that was above his heart shrunk enough for him to resume normal function, he also took his diet into his own hands and worked hard to eat healthy foods and eliminate unhealthy ones. Today, he's healthy, running around and has all his hair back! I hope this book finds you well and if it does not, I hope then this book gives you the tools you need to combat cancer and make your own Road to Remission.

Good luck and all the best with your healthy journey!

Made in the USA
Lexington, KY
09 September 2016